THE 90-DAY
Self-Healing Journal

A GUIDE TO TRANSFORMING YOUR HEALTH INSIDE AND OUT

Discover the power of tracking your physical and mental tendencies to transform your health inside and out by changing your lifestyle, beliefs, and daily habits for the better.

CREATED BY ALEXA FEDERICO, BA, NTP

"And suddenly you know: It's time to start something new and trust the magic of beginnings." - Meister Eckhart

©2019 Alexa Federico
All rights reserved.

Introduction

To the owner of this journal, congratulations! I don't know you, but I do know that you are invested in making your life better and I am here to help with *The 90-Day Self-Healing Journal*. So, why this journal? Through my own years of experience with Crohn's disease (a type of chronic autoimmune illness) and later working with clients to regain their health, I have learned a lot about what it takes to heal.

For years I focused on the physical, tangible parts of healing (like what I was eating, what supplements I was taking, how I was sleeping, etc.) It wasn't until much later when I realized that healing is multi-faceted and includes, without a doubt, the "inner work." It's important to note that everyone's self-healing journey will look very different depending on your past experiences and what's going on currently in your life. Your "inner work" may involve changing your perspective of a situation, instilling new beliefs about yourself, forgiving, as a few examples.

I truly hope this is the start of an eye-opening 90-day journey for you. If this journal has helped you and you'd like to let me know or you just want to say hi, you can contact me by emailing alexa@girlinhealing.com.

In love and light,

Alexa

The Four Pillars of Health

Living a healthy, balanced life is a combination of everything in your life. Your diet, the people in your social circle, the exercise you do, and your views on money are just some examples of what shapes how you feel mentally and physically. I have found that any aspect of life can be filed under one of The Four Pillars of Health. Whether you find yourself feeling "off" or extremely ill, return to the pillars, which are the foundation for health, and reevaluate what could be lacking in your life.

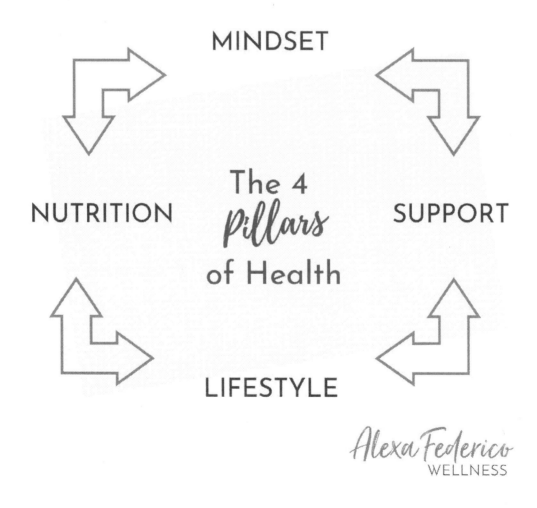

Alexa Federico Wellness

Nutrition

Optimal nutrition gives us more energy, better sleep, less sugar cravings, and so much more. It's our fuel!

Mindset

Perspective is everything. Change the way you view your situation; change your life.

Support

Cultivate a support team who has your back when you need it. Everyone needs help at some point.

Lifestyle

You know bingeing Netflix or feeling dead inside at your job aren't good for you. Now it's time to reflect on what isn't working and what you could add to your routine for a healthier balance.

90-Day Goals

Goal* (*n*): the end toward which effort is directed

As defined by Merriam-Webster

Now, it's time to commit to four goals for the next 90 days; one for each pillar of health. You may know exactly what you want to work on, but you may not, and that's okay! If the latter is true for you, take a few minutes to write out what you currently do for yourself in each pillar and then evaluate where you can improve.

Why make 90-day goals? Many people are used to making yearly goals like:

> "My goal for this year is to go to the gym four times a week."
>
> "My goal for this year is to make six figures."
>
> "My goal for this year is to be more mindful of the amount of time I spend on my phone."

The problem with these is that often people don't sustain the same amount of motivation to work towards their goals for the entire year. At some point, goals start to be "forgotten" about and the individuals that created them in the first place often go back to their past habits.

Through a business lens, 90 days is one quarter, so think of this journal as a place to record, track, and evaluate your goals for one quarter of the year. Just like a company may evaluate their progress on a quarterly basis, you can hold yourself to the same accountability.

Likely, you will see that you might not work on one or two pillars as much as the others. This is completely normal and only strengthens your journal practice. If you find that a goal was not sustainable, you can always come back to this page and adjust your intention. Journaling and goal-setting are practices, so don't be hard on yourself if things don't go perfectly at first.

My nutrition goal for the next 90 days is:

(Examples: Have 2 servings of veggies with every meal. / Add 16oz. to my daily water intake.)

My mindset goal for the next 90 days is:

(Examples: Instead of worrying about what can go wrong, think about what could go right. / Replace negative thoughts about myself with something I love about myself.)

My support goal for the next 90 days is:

(Examples: Meet up with a friend once a week to catch up and enjoy each other's company. / Ask for help instead of trying to do everything on my own.)

My lifestyle goal for the next 90 days is:

(Examples: Go for a walk 3x/week after work for 20-30 minutes. / Wake up 10 minutes earlier to start a morning meditation practice.)

TODAY'S DATE: ___/___/___

QUOTE OF THE DAY:

> "There are many ways of going forward, but only one way of standing still." – Franklin Roosevelt

TODAY I AM GRATEFUL FOR:

DAILY AFFIRMATION:
(WRITE ONCE AND REPEAT THROUGHOUT THE DAY)

> I am always surrounded by love.

NOTES:

FOOD & SYMPTOM TRACKER:

TIME	FOOD	SYMPTOMS & MOOD CHANGES

HOW AM I SUPPORTING EACH OF THE 4 PILLARS OF MY HEALTH?

NUTRITION (NUTRIENT DENSE FOODS, WATER)

LIFESTYLE (SLEEP, STRESS MANAGEMENT, EXERCISE)

MINDSET (AFFIRMATIONS, KIND SELF TALK)

SUPPORT (ASK FOR HELP, REACH OUT TO A FRIEND)

TODAY'S DATE: ___/___/___

QUOTE OF THE DAY:

> *"Failure is not fatal, but failure to change might be."*
> *– John Wooden*

TODAY I AM GRATEFUL FOR:

DAILY AFFIRMATION:
(WRITE ONCE AND REPEAT THROUGHOUT THE DAY)

> *My body is strong and supports me in whatever I desire to do.*

NOTES:

FOOD & SYMPTOM TRACKER:

TIME	FOOD	SYMPTOMS & MOOD CHANGES

HOW AM I SUPPORTING EACH OF THE 4 PILLARS OF MY HEALTH?

NUTRITION (NUTRIENT DENSE FOODS, WATER)

LIFESTYLE (SLEEP, STRESS MANAGEMENT, EXERCISE)

MINDSET (AFFIRMATIONS, KIND SELF TALK)

SUPPORT (ASK FOR HELP, REACH OUT TO A FRIEND)

TODAY'S DATE: ___/___/___

QUOTE OF THE DAY:

"The important thing is not to stop questioning. Curiosity has its own reason for existence..." - Albert Einstein

TODAY I AM GRATEFUL FOR:

DAILY AFFIRMATION:
(WRITE ONCE AND REPEAT THROUGHOUT THE DAY)

I am choosing what feels right in my heart.

NOTES:

FOOD & SYMPTOM TRACKER:

TIME	FOOD	SYMPTOMS & MOOD CHANGES

HOW AM I SUPPORTING EACH OF THE 4 PILLARS OF MY HEALTH?

NUTRITION (NUTRIENT DENSE FOODS, WATER)

LIFESTYLE (SLEEP, STRESS MANAGEMENT, EXERCISE)

MINDSET (AFFIRMATIONS, KIND SELF TALK)

SUPPORT (ASK FOR HELP, REACH OUT TO A FRIEND)

TODAY'S DATE: ___/___/___

QUOTE OF THE DAY:

"Things don't have to change the world to be important."
— Steve Jobs

TODAY I AM GRATEFUL FOR:

DAILY AFFIRMATION:
(WRITE ONCE AND REPEAT THROUGHOUT THE DAY)

More money is always on its way to me.

NOTES:

FOOD & SYMPTOM TRACKER:

TIME	FOOD	SYMPTOMS & MOOD CHANGES

HOW AM I SUPPORTING EACH OF THE 4 PILLARS OF MY HEALTH?

NUTRITION (NUTRIENT DENSE FOODS, WATER)

LIFESTYLE (SLEEP, STRESS MANAGEMENT, EXERCISE)

MINDSET (AFFIRMATIONS, KIND SELF TALK)

SUPPORT (ASK FOR HELP, REACH OUT TO A FRIEND)

TODAY'S DATE: ___/___/___

QUOTE OF THE DAY:

> *"We are all just travelers on one great journey home, in need of daily, grace-filled reminders that none of us are traveling alone." - Morgan Harper Nichols*

TODAY I AM GRATEFUL FOR:

DAILY AFFIRMATION:
(WRITE ONCE AND REPEAT THROUGHOUT THE DAY)

> *I am open to receiving love.*

NOTES:

FOOD & SYMPTOM TRACKER:

TIME	FOOD	SYMPTOMS & MOOD CHANGES

HOW AM I SUPPORTING EACH OF THE 4 PILLARS OF MY HEALTH?

NUTRITION (NUTRIENT DENSE FOODS, WATER)

LIFESTYLE (SLEEP, STRESS MANAGEMENT, EXERCISE)

MINDSET (AFFIRMATIONS, KIND SELF TALK)

SUPPORT (ASK FOR HELP, REACH OUT TO A FRIEND)

TODAY'S DATE: ___/___/___

QUOTE OF THE DAY:

"There are risks and costs to a program of action. But they are far less than the long-range risks and costs of comfortable inaction." - John F. Kennedy

TODAY I AM GRATEFUL FOR:

DAILY AFFIRMATION:
(WRITE ONCE AND REPEAT THROUGHOUT THE DAY)

The right opportunities are coming to me.

NOTES:

FOOD & SYMPTOM TRACKER:

TIME	FOOD	SYMPTOMS & MOOD CHANGES

HOW AM I SUPPORTING EACH OF THE 4 PILLARS OF MY HEALTH?

NUTRITION (NUTRIENT DENSE FOODS, WATER)

LIFESTYLE (SLEEP, STRESS MANAGEMENT, EXERCISE)

MINDSET (AFFIRMATIONS, KIND SELF TALK)

SUPPORT (ASK FOR HELP, REACH OUT TO A FRIEND)

TODAY'S DATE: ___/___/___

QUOTE OF THE DAY:

"Don't look for big things, just do small things with great love." - Mother Teresa

TODAY I AM GRATEFUL FOR:

DAILY AFFIRMATION:
(WRITE ONCE AND REPEAT THROUGHOUT THE DAY)

I experience miracles every day as long as I pay attention.

NOTES:

FOOD & SYMPTOM TRACKER:

TIME	FOOD	SYMPTOMS & MOOD CHANGES

HOW AM I SUPPORTING EACH OF THE 4 PILLARS OF MY HEALTH?

NUTRITION (NUTRIENT DENSE FOODS, WATER)

LIFESTYLE (SLEEP, STRESS MANAGEMENT, EXERCISE)

MINDSET (AFFIRMATIONS, KIND SELF TALK)

SUPPORT (ASK FOR HELP, REACH OUT TO A FRIEND)

TODAY'S DATE: ___/___/___

QUOTE OF THE DAY:

"When you believe in a thing, believe in it all the way, implicitly and unquestionably." – Walt Disney

FOOD & SYMPTOM TRACKER:

TIME	FOOD	SYMPTOMS & MOOD CHANGES

TODAY I AM GRATEFUL FOR:

DAILY AFFIRMATION:
(WRITE ONCE AND REPEAT THROUGHOUT THE DAY)

I am surrounded by people who lift me up.

HOW AM I SUPPORTING EACH OF THE 4 PILLARS OF MY HEALTH?

NUTRITION (NUTRIENT DENSE FOODS, WATER)

LIFESTYLE (SLEEP, STRESS MANAGEMENT, EXERCISE)

MINDSET (AFFIRMATIONS, KIND SELF TALK)

SUPPORT (ASK FOR HELP, REACH OUT TO A FRIEND)

NOTES:

TODAY'S DATE: ___/___/___

QUOTE OF THE DAY:

> "Plant seeds of happiness, hope, success, and love; it will all come back to you in abundance. This is the law of nature."
> — Steve Maraboli

TODAY I AM GRATEFUL FOR:

DAILY AFFIRMATION:
(WRITE ONCE AND REPEAT THROUGHOUT THE DAY)

> New and exciting experiences await me.

NOTES:

FOOD & SYMPTOM TRACKER:

TIME	FOOD	SYMPTOMS & MOOD CHANGES

HOW AM I SUPPORTING EACH OF THE 4 PILLARS OF MY HEALTH?

NUTRITION (NUTRIENT DENSE FOODS, WATER)

LIFESTYLE (SLEEP, STRESS MANAGEMENT, EXERCISE)

MINDSET (AFFIRMATIONS, KIND SELF TALK)

SUPPORT (ASK FOR HELP, REACH OUT TO A FRIEND)

TODAY'S DATE: ___/___/___

QUOTE OF THE DAY:

"Don't surrender all your joy for an idea you used to have about yourself that isn't true anymore." - Cheryl Strayed

TODAY I AM GRATEFUL FOR:

DAILY AFFIRMATION:
(WRITE ONCE AND REPEAT THROUGHOUT THE DAY)

The challenges in my life are teaching me lessons that will make me stronger.

NOTES:

FOOD & SYMPTOM TRACKER:

TIME	FOOD	SYMPTOMS & MOOD CHANGES

HOW AM I SUPPORTING EACH OF THE 4 PILLARS OF MY HEALTH?

NUTRITION (NUTRIENT DENSE FOODS, WATER)

LIFESTYLE (SLEEP, STRESS MANAGEMENT, EXERCISE)

MINDSET (AFFIRMATIONS, KIND SELF TALK)

SUPPORT (ASK FOR HELP, REACH OUT TO A FRIEND)

TODAY'S DATE: ___/___/___

QUOTE OF THE DAY:

> "We can never know how much good a simple smile can do."
> – Mother Teresa

TODAY I AM GRATEFUL FOR:

DAILY AFFIRMATION:
(WRITE ONCE AND REPEAT THROUGHOUT THE DAY)

> I am grateful for waking up today.

NOTES:

FOOD & SYMPTOM TRACKER:

TIME	FOOD	SYMPTOMS & MOOD CHANGES

HOW AM I SUPPORTING EACH OF THE 4 PILLARS OF MY HEALTH?

NUTRITION (NUTRIENT DENSE FOODS, WATER)

LIFESTYLE (SLEEP, STRESS MANAGEMENT, EXERCISE)

MINDSET (AFFIRMATIONS, KIND SELF TALK)

SUPPORT (ASK FOR HELP, REACH OUT TO A FRIEND)

TODAY'S DATE: ___/___/___

QUOTE OF THE DAY:

"You have your way, I have my way. As for the right way, the correct way, and the only way, it does not exist."
— Friedrich Nietzsche

TODAY I AM GRATEFUL FOR:

DAILY AFFIRMATION:
(WRITE ONCE AND REPEAT THROUGHOUT THE DAY)

I am right where I am supposed to be at this point in my life.

NOTES:

FOOD & SYMPTOM TRACKER:

TIME	FOOD	SYMPTOMS & MOOD CHANGES

HOW AM I SUPPORTING EACH OF THE 4 PILLARS OF MY HEALTH?

NUTRITION (NUTRIENT DENSE FOODS, WATER)

LIFESTYLE (SLEEP, STRESS MANAGEMENT, EXERCISE)

MINDSET (AFFIRMATIONS, KIND SELF TALK)

SUPPORT (ASK FOR HELP, REACH OUT TO A FRIEND)

TODAY'S DATE: ___/___/___

QUOTE OF THE DAY:

> *"If we are together, nothing is impossible. If we are divided, all will fail."* – Winston Churchill

TODAY I AM GRATEFUL FOR:

DAILY AFFIRMATION:
(WRITE ONCE AND REPEAT THROUGHOUT THE DAY)

> *Sleep comes easily to me and I wake up restful.*

NOTES:

FOOD & SYMPTOM TRACKER:

TIME	FOOD	SYMPTOMS & MOOD CHANGES

HOW AM I SUPPORTING EACH OF THE 4 PILLARS OF MY HEALTH?

NUTRITION (NUTRIENT DENSE FOODS, WATER)

LIFESTYLE (SLEEP, STRESS MANAGEMENT, EXERCISE)

MINDSET (AFFIRMATIONS, KIND SELF TALK)

SUPPORT (ASK FOR HELP, REACH OUT TO A FRIEND)

TODAY'S DATE: ___/___/___

QUOTE OF THE DAY:

> *"The most common way people give up their power is by thinking they don't have any."* — Alice Walker

TODAY I AM GRATEFUL FOR:

DAILY AFFIRMATION:
(WRITE ONCE AND REPEAT THROUGHOUT THE DAY)

> *I exude confidence in the way I walk, talk, and live.*

NOTES:

FOOD & SYMPTOM TRACKER:

TIME	FOOD	SYMPTOMS & MOOD CHANGES

HOW AM I SUPPORTING EACH OF THE 4 PILLARS OF MY HEALTH?

NUTRITION (NUTRIENT DENSE FOODS, WATER)

LIFESTYLE (SLEEP, STRESS MANAGEMENT, EXERCISE)

MINDSET (AFFIRMATIONS, KIND SELF TALK)

SUPPORT (ASK FOR HELP, REACH OUT TO A FRIEND)

TODAY'S DATE: ___/___/___

QUOTE OF THE DAY:

"Once you have established the goals you want and the price you're willing to pay, you can ignore the minor hurts, the opponent's pressure, and the temporary failures." - Vince Lombardi

TODAY I AM GRATEFUL FOR:

DAILY AFFIRMATION:
(WRITE ONCE AND REPEAT THROUGHOUT THE DAY)

I keep the promises I make to myself and others.

NOTES:

FOOD & SYMPTOM TRACKER:

TIME	FOOD	SYMPTOMS & MOOD CHANGES

HOW AM I SUPPORTING EACH OF THE 4 PILLARS OF MY HEALTH?

NUTRITION (NUTRIENT DENSE FOODS, WATER)

LIFESTYLE (SLEEP, STRESS MANAGEMENT, EXERCISE)

MINDSET (AFFIRMATIONS, KIND SELF TALK)

SUPPORT (ASK FOR HELP, REACH OUT TO A FRIEND)

TODAY'S DATE: ___/___/___

QUOTE OF THE DAY:

> "I cannot discover that anyone knows enough to say definitely what is and what is not possible." – Henry Ford

TODAY I AM GRATEFUL FOR:

DAILY AFFIRMATION:
(WRITE ONCE AND REPEAT THROUGHOUT THE DAY)

> I have control of the choices I make in life.

NOTES:

FOOD & SYMPTOM TRACKER:

TIME	FOOD	SYMPTOMS & MOOD CHANGES

HOW AM I SUPPORTING EACH OF THE 4 PILLARS OF MY HEALTH?

NUTRITION (NUTRIENT DENSE FOODS, WATER)

LIFESTYLE (SLEEP, STRESS MANAGEMENT, EXERCISE)

MINDSET (AFFIRMATIONS, KIND SELF TALK)

SUPPORT (ASK FOR HELP, REACH OUT TO A FRIEND)

TODAY'S DATE: ___/___/___

QUOTE OF THE DAY:

"There is no passion to be found playing small—in settling for a life that is less than the one you are capable of living."
— Nelson Mandela

FOOD & SYMPTOM TRACKER:

TIME	FOOD	SYMPTOMS & MOOD CHANGES

TODAY I AM GRATEFUL FOR:

DAILY AFFIRMATION:
(WRITE ONCE AND REPEAT THROUGHOUT THE DAY)

I choose to be happy today.

HOW AM I SUPPORTING EACH OF THE 4 PILLARS OF MY HEALTH?

NUTRITION (NUTRIENT DENSE FOODS, WATER)

LIFESTYLE (SLEEP, STRESS MANAGEMENT, EXERCISE)

MINDSET (AFFIRMATIONS, KIND SELF TALK)

SUPPORT (ASK FOR HELP, REACH OUT TO A FRIEND)

NOTES:

TODAY'S DATE: ___/___/___

QUOTE OF THE DAY:

"Traveler, there is no path, the path must be forged as you walk."
— Antonio Machado

TODAY I AM GRATEFUL FOR:

DAILY AFFIRMATION:
(WRITE ONCE AND REPEAT THROUGHOUT THE DAY)

Everything happens for me, not to me.

NOTES:

FOOD & SYMPTOM TRACKER:

TIME	FOOD	SYMPTOMS & MOOD CHANGES

HOW AM I SUPPORTING EACH OF THE 4 PILLARS OF MY HEALTH?

NUTRITION (NUTRIENT DENSE FOODS, WATER)

LIFESTYLE (SLEEP, STRESS MANAGEMENT, EXERCISE)

MINDSET (AFFIRMATIONS, KIND SELF TALK)

SUPPORT (ASK FOR HELP, REACH OUT TO A FRIEND)

TODAY'S DATE: ___/___/___

QUOTE OF THE DAY:

"Life is one grand, sweet song, so start the music."
— *Ronald Regan*

TODAY I AM GRATEFUL FOR:

DAILY AFFIRMATION:
(WRITE ONCE AND REPEAT THROUGHOUT THE DAY)

I am capable of creating the best life I can imagine.

NOTES:

FOOD & SYMPTOM TRACKER:

TIME	FOOD	SYMPTOMS & MOOD CHANGES

HOW AM I SUPPORTING EACH OF THE 4 PILLARS OF MY HEALTH?

NUTRITION (NUTRIENT DENSE FOODS, WATER)

LIFESTYLE (SLEEP, STRESS MANAGEMENT, EXERCISE)

MINDSET (AFFIRMATIONS, KIND SELF TALK)

SUPPORT (ASK FOR HELP, REACH OUT TO A FRIEND)

TODAY'S DATE: ___/___/___

QUOTE OF THE DAY:

"We are what we repeatedly do. Excellence, then, is not an act, but a habit." – Aristotle

TODAY I AM GRATEFUL FOR:

DAILY AFFIRMATION:
(WRITE ONCE AND REPEAT THROUGHOUT THE DAY)

When my gut tells me something is off, I listen to my intuition.

NOTES:

FOOD & SYMPTOM TRACKER:

TIME	FOOD	SYMPTOMS & MOOD CHANGES

HOW AM I SUPPORTING EACH OF THE 4 PILLARS OF MY HEALTH?

NUTRITION (NUTRIENT DENSE FOODS, WATER)

LIFESTYLE (SLEEP, STRESS MANAGEMENT, EXERCISE)

MINDSET (AFFIRMATIONS, KIND SELF TALK)

SUPPORT (ASK FOR HELP, REACH OUT TO A FRIEND)

TODAY'S DATE: ___/___/___

QUOTE OF THE DAY:

"Take time for all things: great haste makes great waste."
— Benjamin Franklin

TODAY I AM GRATEFUL FOR:

DAILY AFFIRMATION:
(WRITE ONCE AND REPEAT THROUGHOUT THE DAY)

I surround myself with people who "get" me.

NOTES:

FOOD & SYMPTOM TRACKER:

TIME	FOOD	SYMPTOMS & MOOD CHANGES

HOW AM I SUPPORTING EACH OF THE 4 PILLARS OF MY HEALTH?

NUTRITION (NUTRIENT DENSE FOODS, WATER)

LIFESTYLE (SLEEP, STRESS MANAGEMENT, EXERCISE)

MINDSET (AFFIRMATIONS, KIND SELF TALK)

SUPPORT (ASK FOR HELP, REACH OUT TO A FRIEND)

TODAY'S DATE: ___/___/___

QUOTE OF THE DAY:

> *"You don't get what you want. You get your unconscious habits."*
> *— Jim Fortin*

TODAY I AM GRATEFUL FOR:

DAILY AFFIRMATION:
(WRITE ONCE AND REPEAT THROUGHOUT THE DAY)

> *Every day I do at least one thing that brings me joy.*

NOTES:

FOOD & SYMPTOM TRACKER:

TIME	FOOD	SYMPTOMS & MOOD CHANGES

HOW AM I SUPPORTING EACH OF THE 4 PILLARS OF MY HEALTH?

NUTRITION (NUTRIENT DENSE FOODS, WATER)

LIFESTYLE (SLEEP, STRESS MANAGEMENT, EXERCISE)

MINDSET (AFFIRMATIONS, KIND SELF TALK)

SUPPORT (ASK FOR HELP, REACH OUT TO A FRIEND)

TODAY'S DATE: ___/___/___

QUOTE OF THE DAY:

"A man is but the products of his thoughts. What he thinks, he becomes." – Mahatma Gandhi

TODAY I AM GRATEFUL FOR:

DAILY AFFIRMATION:
(WRITE ONCE AND REPEAT THROUGHOUT THE DAY)

I love money and all that it does for me. I am always receiving more!

NOTES:

FOOD & SYMPTOM TRACKER:

TIME	FOOD	SYMPTOMS & MOOD CHANGES

HOW AM I SUPPORTING EACH OF THE 4 PILLARS OF MY HEALTH?

NUTRITION (NUTRIENT DENSE FOODS, WATER)

LIFESTYLE (SLEEP, STRESS MANAGEMENT, EXERCISE)

MINDSET (AFFIRMATIONS, KIND SELF TALK)

SUPPORT (ASK FOR HELP, REACH OUT TO A FRIEND)

TODAY'S DATE: ___/___/___

QUOTE OF THE DAY:

"Trouble knocked at the door, but, hearing laughter, hurried away."
- Benjamin Franklin

TODAY I AM GRATEFUL FOR:

DAILY AFFIRMATION:
(WRITE ONCE AND REPEAT THROUGHOUT THE DAY)

I am worthy of the love I wish for other people.

NOTES:

FOOD & SYMPTOM TRACKER:

TIME	FOOD	SYMPTOMS & MOOD CHANGES

HOW AM I SUPPORTING EACH OF THE 4 PILLARS OF MY HEALTH?

NUTRITION (NUTRIENT DENSE FOODS, WATER)

LIFESTYLE (SLEEP, STRESS MANAGEMENT, EXERCISE)

MINDSET (AFFIRMATIONS, KIND SELF TALK)

SUPPORT (ASK FOR HELP, REACH OUT TO A FRIEND)

TODAY'S DATE: ___/___/___

QUOTE OF THE DAY:

"Do what you can, with what you have, where you are."
— Theodore Roosevelt

TODAY I AM GRATEFUL FOR:

DAILY AFFIRMATION:
(WRITE ONCE AND REPEAT THROUGHOUT THE DAY)

I have patience with myself when I am struggling.

NOTES:

FOOD & SYMPTOM TRACKER:

TIME	FOOD	SYMPTOMS & MOOD CHANGES

HOW AM I SUPPORTING EACH OF THE 4 PILLARS OF MY HEALTH?

NUTRITION (NUTRIENT DENSE FOODS, WATER)

LIFESTYLE (SLEEP, STRESS MANAGEMENT, EXERCISE)

MINDSET (AFFIRMATIONS, KIND SELF TALK)

SUPPORT (ASK FOR HELP, REACH OUT TO A FRIEND)

TODAY'S DATE: ___/___/___

QUOTE OF THE DAY:

> "Take time to deliberate; but when the time for action arrives, stop thinking and go in." - Andrew Jackson

TODAY I AM GRATEFUL FOR:

DAILY AFFIRMATION:
(WRITE ONCE AND REPEAT THROUGHOUT THE DAY)

> I am divinely perfect the exact way that I am.

NOTES:

FOOD & SYMPTOM TRACKER:

TIME	FOOD	SYMPTOMS & MOOD CHANGES

HOW AM I SUPPORTING EACH OF THE 4 PILLARS OF MY HEALTH?

NUTRITION (NUTRIENT DENSE FOODS, WATER)

LIFESTYLE (SLEEP, STRESS MANAGEMENT, EXERCISE)

MINDSET (AFFIRMATIONS, KIND SELF TALK)

SUPPORT (ASK FOR HELP, REACH OUT TO A FRIEND)

TODAY'S DATE: ___/___/___

QUOTE OF THE DAY:

"Embrace who you are. Literally. Hug yourself. Accept who you are."
- Ellen DeGeneres

TODAY I AM GRATEFUL FOR:

DAILY AFFIRMATION:
(WRITE ONCE AND REPEAT THROUGHOUT THE DAY)

I forgive those who have hurt me and free myself from their burden.

NOTES:

FOOD & SYMPTOM TRACKER:

TIME	FOOD	SYMPTOMS & MOOD CHANGES

HOW AM I SUPPORTING EACH OF THE 4 PILLARS OF MY HEALTH?

NUTRITION (NUTRIENT DENSE FOODS, WATER)

LIFESTYLE (SLEEP, STRESS MANAGEMENT, EXERCISE)

MINDSET (AFFIRMATIONS, KIND SELF TALK)

SUPPORT (ASK FOR HELP, REACH OUT TO A FRIEND)

TODAY'S DATE: ___/___/___

QUOTE OF THE DAY:

"She will not worry, she will be just fine. She will brave the new season one day at a time." – Morgan Harper Nichols

TODAY I AM GRATEFUL FOR:

DAILY AFFIRMATION:
(WRITE ONCE AND REPEAT THROUGHOUT THE DAY)

My life is full and abundant and I experience joy every day.

NOTES:

FOOD & SYMPTOM TRACKER:

TIME	FOOD	SYMPTOMS & MOOD CHANGES

HOW AM I SUPPORTING EACH OF THE 4 PILLARS OF MY HEALTH?

NUTRITION (NUTRIENT DENSE FOODS, WATER)

LIFESTYLE (SLEEP, STRESS MANAGEMENT, EXERCISE)

MINDSET (AFFIRMATIONS, KIND SELF TALK)

SUPPORT (ASK FOR HELP, REACH OUT TO A FRIEND)

TODAY'S DATE: ___/___/___

QUOTE OF THE DAY:

> "You are going to live a good and long life filled with great and terrible moments that you cannot even imagine yet." – John Green

TODAY I AM GRATEFUL FOR:

DAILY AFFIRMATION:
(WRITE ONCE AND REPEAT THROUGHOUT THE DAY)

> Today I will ask for help when things feel heavy.

NOTES:

FOOD & SYMPTOM TRACKER:

TIME	FOOD	SYMPTOMS & MOOD CHANGES

HOW AM I SUPPORTING EACH OF THE 4 PILLARS OF MY HEALTH?

NUTRITION (NUTRIENT DENSE FOODS, WATER)

LIFESTYLE (SLEEP, STRESS MANAGEMENT, EXERCISE)

MINDSET (AFFIRMATIONS, KIND SELF TALK)

SUPPORT (ASK FOR HELP, REACH OUT TO A FRIEND)

TODAY'S DATE: ___/___/___

QUOTE OF THE DAY:

"Even if your ambitions are huge, start slow, start small, build gradually, build smart." – Gary Vaynerchuk

TODAY I AM GRATEFUL FOR:

DAILY AFFIRMATION:
(WRITE ONCE AND REPEAT THROUGHOUT THE DAY)

Money allows me to eat, sleep, travel, and live well. I am so grateful for money.

NOTES:

FOOD & SYMPTOM TRACKER:

TIME	FOOD	SYMPTOMS & MOOD CHANGES

HOW AM I SUPPORTING EACH OF THE 4 PILLARS OF MY HEALTH?

NUTRITION (NUTRIENT DENSE FOODS, WATER)

LIFESTYLE (SLEEP, STRESS MANAGEMENT, EXERCISE)

MINDSET (AFFIRMATIONS, KIND SELF TALK)

SUPPORT (ASK FOR HELP, REACH OUT TO A FRIEND)

TODAY'S DATE: ___/___/___

QUOTE OF THE DAY:

"What makes night within us may leave stars."
– Victor Hugo

TODAY I AM GRATEFUL FOR:

DAILY AFFIRMATION:
(WRITE ONCE AND REPEAT THROUGHOUT THE DAY)

My value is based on who I am and how I treat others, not on materialistic things.

NOTES:

FOOD & SYMPTOM TRACKER:

TIME	FOOD	SYMPTOMS & MOOD CHANGES

HOW AM I SUPPORTING EACH OF THE 4 PILLARS OF MY HEALTH?

NUTRITION (NUTRIENT DENSE FOODS, WATER)

LIFESTYLE (SLEEP, STRESS MANAGEMENT, EXERCISE)

MINDSET (AFFIRMATIONS, KIND SELF TALK)

SUPPORT (ASK FOR HELP, REACH OUT TO A FRIEND)

TODAY'S DATE: ___/___/___

QUOTE OF THE DAY:

> "One of the greatest discoveries a man makes, one of his great surprises, is to find he can do what he was afraid he couldn't do." – Henry Ford

TODAY I AM GRATEFUL FOR:

DAILY AFFIRMATION:
(WRITE ONCE AND REPEAT THROUGHOUT THE DAY)

> Positive energy flows freely to me.

NOTES:

FOOD & SYMPTOM TRACKER:

TIME	FOOD	SYMPTOMS & MOOD CHANGES

HOW AM I SUPPORTING EACH OF THE 4 PILLARS OF MY HEALTH?

NUTRITION (NUTRIENT DENSE FOODS, WATER)

LIFESTYLE (SLEEP, STRESS MANAGEMENT, EXERCISE)

MINDSET (AFFIRMATIONS, KIND SELF TALK)

SUPPORT (ASK FOR HELP, REACH OUT TO A FRIEND)

TODAY'S DATE: ___/___/___

QUOTE OF THE DAY:

"My own prescription for health is less paperwork and more running barefoot through the grass." - Leslie Grimutter

TODAY I AM GRATEFUL FOR:

DAILY AFFIRMATION:
(WRITE ONCE AND REPEAT THROUGHOUT THE DAY)

I am always learning and growing mentally and spiritually.

NOTES:

FOOD & SYMPTOM TRACKER:

TIME	FOOD	SYMPTOMS & MOOD CHANGES

HOW AM I SUPPORTING EACH OF THE 4 PILLARS OF MY HEALTH?

NUTRITION (NUTRIENT DENSE FOODS, WATER)

LIFESTYLE (SLEEP, STRESS MANAGEMENT, EXERCISE)

MINDSET (AFFIRMATIONS, KIND SELF TALK)

SUPPORT (ASK FOR HELP, REACH OUT TO A FRIEND)

TODAY'S DATE: ___/___/___

QUOTE OF THE DAY:

"Have patience with everything that remains unresolved in your heart." – Rainer Maria Rilke

TODAY I AM GRATEFUL FOR:

DAILY AFFIRMATION:
(WRITE ONCE AND REPEAT THROUGHOUT THE DAY)

*I trust the flow of my life.
I am on the right track.*

NOTES:

FOOD & SYMPTOM TRACKER:

TIME	FOOD	SYMPTOMS & MOOD CHANGES

HOW AM I SUPPORTING EACH OF THE 4 PILLARS OF MY HEALTH?

NUTRITION (NUTRIENT DENSE FOODS, WATER)

LIFESTYLE (SLEEP, STRESS MANAGEMENT, EXERCISE)

MINDSET (AFFIRMATIONS, KIND SELF TALK)

SUPPORT (ASK FOR HELP, REACH OUT TO A FRIEND)

TODAY'S DATE: ___/___/___

QUOTE OF THE DAY:

"Just to breathe is enough to always be happy, to always be in love." – Don Miguel Ruiz

TODAY I AM GRATEFUL FOR:

DAILY AFFIRMATION:
(WRITE ONCE AND REPEAT THROUGHOUT THE DAY)

My efforts are admired and appreciated.

NOTES:

FOOD & SYMPTOM TRACKER:

TIME	FOOD	SYMPTOMS & MOOD CHANGES

HOW AM I SUPPORTING EACH OF THE 4 PILLARS OF MY HEALTH?

NUTRITION (NUTRIENT DENSE FOODS, WATER)

LIFESTYLE (SLEEP, STRESS MANAGEMENT, EXERCISE)

MINDSET (AFFIRMATIONS, KIND SELF TALK)

SUPPORT (ASK FOR HELP, REACH OUT TO A FRIEND)

TODAY'S DATE: ___/___/___

QUOTE OF THE DAY:

"Do not let what you cannot do interfere with what you can do."
– John Wooden

TODAY I AM GRATEFUL FOR:

DAILY AFFIRMATION:
(WRITE ONCE AND REPEAT THROUGHOUT THE DAY)

I am overflowing with love and compassion for others.

NOTES:

FOOD & SYMPTOM TRACKER:

TIME	FOOD	SYMPTOMS & MOOD CHANGES

HOW AM I SUPPORTING EACH OF THE 4 PILLARS OF MY HEALTH?

NUTRITION (NUTRIENT DENSE FOODS, WATER)

LIFESTYLE (SLEEP, STRESS MANAGEMENT, EXERCISE)

MINDSET (AFFIRMATIONS, KIND SELF TALK)

SUPPORT (ASK FOR HELP, REACH OUT TO A FRIEND)

TODAY'S DATE: ___/___/___

QUOTE OF THE DAY:

"The best and most beautiful things in the world cannot be seen or even touched—they must be felt with the heart." - Helen Keller

TODAY I AM GRATEFUL FOR:

DAILY AFFIRMATION:
(WRITE ONCE AND REPEAT THROUGHOUT THE DAY)

I welcome new friends and connections into my life.

NOTES:

FOOD & SYMPTOM TRACKER:

TIME	FOOD	SYMPTOMS & MOOD CHANGES

HOW AM I SUPPORTING EACH OF THE 4 PILLARS OF MY HEALTH?

NUTRITION (NUTRIENT DENSE FOODS, WATER)

LIFESTYLE (SLEEP, STRESS MANAGEMENT, EXERCISE)

MINDSET (AFFIRMATIONS, KIND SELF TALK)

SUPPORT (ASK FOR HELP, REACH OUT TO A FRIEND)

TODAY'S DATE: ___/___/___

QUOTE OF THE DAY:

> "How wonderful it is that nobody need wait a single moment before starting to improve the world." – Anne Frank

TODAY I AM GRATEFUL FOR:

DAILY AFFIRMATION:
(WRITE ONCE AND REPEAT THROUGHOUT THE DAY)

> I am committed to prioritizing my happiness and health.

NOTES:

FOOD & SYMPTOM TRACKER:

TIME	FOOD	SYMPTOMS & MOOD CHANGES

HOW AM I SUPPORTING EACH OF THE 4 PILLARS OF MY HEALTH?

NUTRITION (NUTRIENT DENSE FOODS, WATER)

LIFESTYLE (SLEEP, STRESS MANAGEMENT, EXERCISE)

MINDSET (AFFIRMATIONS, KIND SELF TALK)

SUPPORT (ASK FOR HELP, REACH OUT TO A FRIEND)

TODAY'S DATE: ___/___/___

QUOTE OF THE DAY:

> *"Never go to sleep without a request to your subconscious."*
> *— Thomas Edison*

TODAY I AM GRATEFUL FOR:

DAILY AFFIRMATION:
(WRITE ONCE AND REPEAT THROUGHOUT THE DAY)

> *I radiate light to everyone around me.*

NOTES:

FOOD & SYMPTOM TRACKER:

TIME	FOOD	SYMPTOMS & MOOD CHANGES

HOW AM I SUPPORTING EACH OF THE 4 PILLARS OF MY HEALTH?

NUTRITION (NUTRIENT DENSE FOODS, WATER)

LIFESTYLE (SLEEP, STRESS MANAGEMENT, EXERCISE)

MINDSET (AFFIRMATIONS, KIND SELF TALK)

SUPPORT (ASK FOR HELP, REACH OUT TO A FRIEND)

TODAY'S DATE: ___/___/___

QUOTE OF THE DAY:

"Give every day the chance to become the most beautiful of your life."
— Mark Twain

TODAY I AM GRATEFUL FOR:

DAILY AFFIRMATION:
(WRITE ONCE AND REPEAT THROUGHOUT THE DAY)

I am at peace.

NOTES:

FOOD & SYMPTOM TRACKER:

TIME	FOOD	SYMPTOMS & MOOD CHANGES

HOW AM I SUPPORTING EACH OF THE 4 PILLARS OF MY HEALTH?

NUTRITION (NUTRIENT DENSE FOODS, WATER)

LIFESTYLE (SLEEP, STRESS MANAGEMENT, EXERCISE)

MINDSET (AFFIRMATIONS, KIND SELF TALK)

SUPPORT (ASK FOR HELP, REACH OUT TO A FRIEND)

TODAY'S DATE: ___/___/___

QUOTE OF THE DAY:

> "Live in the sunshine, swim the sea, drink the wild air."
> – Ralph Waldo Emerson

TODAY I AM GRATEFUL FOR:

DAILY AFFIRMATION:
(WRITE ONCE AND REPEAT THROUGHOUT THE DAY)

> I trust my intuition to guide my decision-making.

NOTES:

FOOD & SYMPTOM TRACKER:

TIME	FOOD	SYMPTOMS & MOOD CHANGES

HOW AM I SUPPORTING EACH OF THE 4 PILLARS OF MY HEALTH?

NUTRITION (NUTRIENT DENSE FOODS, WATER)

LIFESTYLE (SLEEP, STRESS MANAGEMENT, EXERCISE)

MINDSET (AFFIRMATIONS, KIND SELF TALK)

SUPPORT (ASK FOR HELP, REACH OUT TO A FRIEND)

TODAY'S DATE: ___/___/___

QUOTE OF THE DAY:

*"I am the master of my fate:
I am the captain of my soul."
- William Ernest Henley*

TODAY I AM GRATEFUL FOR:

DAILY AFFIRMATION:
(WRITE ONCE AND REPEAT THROUGHOUT THE DAY)

I attract people who have my best intentions at heart.

NOTES:

FOOD & SYMPTOM TRACKER:

TIME	FOOD	SYMPTOMS & MOOD CHANGES

HOW AM I SUPPORTING EACH OF THE 4 PILLARS OF MY HEALTH?

NUTRITION (NUTRIENT DENSE FOODS, WATER)

LIFESTYLE (SLEEP, STRESS MANAGEMENT, EXERCISE)

MINDSET (AFFIRMATIONS, KIND SELF TALK)

SUPPORT (ASK FOR HELP, REACH OUT TO A FRIEND)

TODAY'S DATE: ___/___/___

QUOTE OF THE DAY:

> "The life you have led doesn't need to be the only life you have."
> – Anna Quindlen

TODAY I AM GRATEFUL FOR:

DAILY AFFIRMATION:
(WRITE ONCE AND REPEAT THROUGHOUT THE DAY)

> I am fully healed.

NOTES:

FOOD & SYMPTOM TRACKER:

TIME	FOOD	SYMPTOMS & MOOD CHANGES

HOW AM I SUPPORTING EACH OF THE 4 PILLARS OF MY HEALTH?

NUTRITION (NUTRIENT DENSE FOODS, WATER)

LIFESTYLE (SLEEP, STRESS MANAGEMENT, EXERCISE)

MINDSET (AFFIRMATIONS, KIND SELF TALK)

SUPPORT (ASK FOR HELP, REACH OUT TO A FRIEND)

TODAY'S DATE: ___/___/___

QUOTE OF THE DAY:

"You learn a lot about someone when you share a meal together."
- Anthony Bourdain

TODAY I AM GRATEFUL FOR:

DAILY AFFIRMATION:
(WRITE ONCE AND REPEAT THROUGHOUT THE DAY)

I take great care of my body because it is my home.

NOTES:

FOOD & SYMPTOM TRACKER:

TIME	FOOD	SYMPTOMS & MOOD CHANGES

HOW AM I SUPPORTING EACH OF THE 4 PILLARS OF MY HEALTH?

NUTRITION (NUTRIENT DENSE FOODS, WATER)

LIFESTYLE (SLEEP, STRESS MANAGEMENT, EXERCISE)

MINDSET (AFFIRMATIONS, KIND SELF TALK)

SUPPORT (ASK FOR HELP, REACH OUT TO A FRIEND)

TODAY'S DATE: ___/___/___

QUOTE OF THE DAY:

> *"You don't become what you want, you become what you believe."* - Oprah

TODAY I AM GRATEFUL FOR:

DAILY AFFIRMATION:
(WRITE ONCE AND REPEAT THROUGHOUT THE DAY)

> *I do things daily that nourish my soul.*

NOTES:

FOOD & SYMPTOM TRACKER:

TIME	FOOD	SYMPTOMS & MOOD CHANGES

HOW AM I SUPPORTING EACH OF THE 4 PILLARS OF MY HEALTH?

NUTRITION (NUTRIENT DENSE FOODS, WATER)

LIFESTYLE (SLEEP, STRESS MANAGEMENT, EXERCISE)

MINDSET (AFFIRMATIONS, KIND SELF TALK)

SUPPORT (ASK FOR HELP, REACH OUT TO A FRIEND)

TODAY'S DATE: ___/___/___

QUOTE OF THE DAY:

"In the depths of winter I finally learned there was in me an invincible summer." - Albert Camus

TODAY I AM GRATEFUL FOR:

DAILY AFFIRMATION:
(WRITE ONCE AND REPEAT THROUGHOUT THE DAY)

I love to move my body because it can do amazing things.

NOTES:

FOOD & SYMPTOM TRACKER:

TIME	FOOD	SYMPTOMS & MOOD CHANGES

HOW AM I SUPPORTING EACH OF THE 4 PILLARS OF MY HEALTH?

NUTRITION (NUTRIENT DENSE FOODS, WATER)

LIFESTYLE (SLEEP, STRESS MANAGEMENT, EXERCISE)

MINDSET (AFFIRMATIONS, KIND SELF TALK)

SUPPORT (ASK FOR HELP, REACH OUT TO A FRIEND)

TODAY'S DATE: ___/___/___

QUOTE OF THE DAY:

> *"We don't create abundance. Abundance is always present. We create limitations."* – James Wedmore

TODAY I AM GRATEFUL FOR:

DAILY AFFIRMATION:
(WRITE ONCE AND REPEAT THROUGHOUT THE DAY)

> *There is something to learn from every experience I have.*

NOTES:

FOOD & SYMPTOM TRACKER:

TIME	FOOD	SYMPTOMS & MOOD CHANGES

HOW AM I SUPPORTING EACH OF THE 4 PILLARS OF MY HEALTH?

NUTRITION (NUTRIENT DENSE FOODS, WATER)

LIFESTYLE (SLEEP, STRESS MANAGEMENT, EXERCISE)

MINDSET (AFFIRMATIONS, KIND SELF TALK)

SUPPORT (ASK FOR HELP, REACH OUT TO A FRIEND)

TODAY'S DATE: ___/___/___

QUOTE OF THE DAY:

"It's up to us to choose contentment and thankfulness now—and to stop imagining that we have to have everything perfect before we'll be happy." - Joanna Gaines

TODAY I AM GRATEFUL FOR:

DAILY AFFIRMATION:
(WRITE ONCE AND REPEAT THROUGHOUT THE DAY)

I love myself even when I am making mistakes.

NOTES:

FOOD & SYMPTOM TRACKER:

TIME	FOOD	SYMPTOMS & MOOD CHANGES

HOW AM I SUPPORTING EACH OF THE 4 PILLARS OF MY HEALTH?

NUTRITION (NUTRIENT DENSE FOODS, WATER)

LIFESTYLE (SLEEP, STRESS MANAGEMENT, EXERCISE)

MINDSET (AFFIRMATIONS, KIND SELF TALK)

SUPPORT (ASK FOR HELP, REACH OUT TO A FRIEND)

TODAY'S DATE: ___/___/___

QUOTE OF THE DAY:

> "Have no fear, you will find your way. It's in your bones. It's in your soul." – Mark Z. Danielewski

TODAY I AM GRATEFUL FOR:

DAILY AFFIRMATION:
(WRITE ONCE AND REPEAT THROUGHOUT THE DAY)

> Every person who comes into my life serves a purpose.

NOTES:

FOOD & SYMPTOM TRACKER:

TIME	FOOD	SYMPTOMS & MOOD CHANGES

HOW AM I SUPPORTING EACH OF THE 4 PILLARS OF MY HEALTH?

NUTRITION (NUTRIENT DENSE FOODS, WATER)

LIFESTYLE (SLEEP, STRESS MANAGEMENT, EXERCISE)

MINDSET (AFFIRMATIONS, KIND SELF TALK)

SUPPORT (ASK FOR HELP, REACH OUT TO A FRIEND)

TODAY'S DATE: ___/___/___

QUOTE OF THE DAY:

"Always keep your eyes open. Keep watching. Because whatever you see can inspire you." – Grace Coddington

TODAY I AM GRATEFUL FOR:

FOOD & SYMPTOM TRACKER:

TIME	FOOD	SYMPTOMS & MOOD CHANGES

DAILY AFFIRMATION:
(WRITE ONCE AND REPEAT THROUGHOUT THE DAY)

I am manifesting my dreams every day.

HOW AM I SUPPORTING EACH OF THE 4 PILLARS OF MY HEALTH?

NUTRITION (NUTRIENT DENSE FOODS, WATER)

LIFESTYLE (SLEEP, STRESS MANAGEMENT, EXERCISE)

MINDSET (AFFIRMATIONS, KIND SELF TALK)

SUPPORT (ASK FOR HELP, REACH OUT TO A FRIEND)

NOTES:

TODAY'S DATE: ___/___/___

QUOTE OF THE DAY:

> "...Be strong, trust yourself, love yourself. Conquer your fears. Just go after what you want and act fast, because life just isn't that long." - Pam Beasley in "The Office"

TODAY I AM GRATEFUL FOR:

DAILY AFFIRMATION:
(WRITE ONCE AND REPEAT THROUGHOUT THE DAY)

> There are an unlimited number of things to be grateful for every single day.

NOTES:

FOOD & SYMPTOM TRACKER:

TIME	FOOD	SYMPTOMS & MOOD CHANGES

HOW AM I SUPPORTING EACH OF THE 4 PILLARS OF MY HEALTH?

NUTRITION (NUTRIENT DENSE FOODS, WATER)

LIFESTYLE (SLEEP, STRESS MANAGEMENT, EXERCISE)

MINDSET (AFFIRMATIONS, KIND SELF TALK)

SUPPORT (ASK FOR HELP, REACH OUT TO A FRIEND)

TODAY'S DATE: ___/___/___

QUOTE OF THE DAY:

"You either walk inside your story and own it or you stand outside your story and hustle for your worthiness."
— Brené Brown

TODAY I AM GRATEFUL FOR:

DAILY AFFIRMATION:
(WRITE ONCE AND REPEAT THROUGHOUT THE DAY)

I am grateful for my job and the security it brings.

NOTES:

FOOD & SYMPTOM TRACKER:

TIME	FOOD	SYMPTOMS & MOOD CHANGES

HOW AM I SUPPORTING EACH OF THE 4 PILLARS OF MY HEALTH?

NUTRITION (NUTRIENT DENSE FOODS, WATER)

LIFESTYLE (SLEEP, STRESS MANAGEMENT, EXERCISE)

MINDSET (AFFIRMATIONS, KIND SELF TALK)

SUPPORT (ASK FOR HELP, REACH OUT TO A FRIEND)

TODAY'S DATE: ___/___/___

QUOTE OF THE DAY:

"And by the way, everything in life is writable about if you have the outgoing guts to do it, and the imagination to improvise. The worst enemy to creativity is self-doubt."
— Sylvia Plath

TODAY I AM GRATEFUL FOR:

DAILY AFFIRMATION:
(WRITE ONCE AND REPEAT THROUGHOUT THE DAY)

I am full of energy and liveliness.

NOTES:

FOOD & SYMPTOM TRACKER:

TIME	FOOD	SYMPTOMS & MOOD CHANGES

HOW AM I SUPPORTING EACH OF THE 4 PILLARS OF MY HEALTH?

NUTRITION (NUTRIENT DENSE FOODS, WATER)

LIFESTYLE (SLEEP, STRESS MANAGEMENT, EXERCISE)

MINDSET (AFFIRMATIONS, KIND SELF TALK)

SUPPORT (ASK FOR HELP, REACH OUT TO A FRIEND)

TODAY'S DATE: ___/___/___

QUOTE OF THE DAY:

> *"There is no way to happiness. Happiness is the way."*
> *— Thich Nhat Hanh*

TODAY I AM GRATEFUL FOR:

DAILY AFFIRMATION:
(WRITE ONCE AND REPEAT THROUGHOUT THE DAY)

> *Today I will check in with myself to make sure my mental and emotional needs are being met.*

NOTES:

FOOD & SYMPTOM TRACKER:

TIME	FOOD	SYMPTOMS & MOOD CHANGES

HOW AM I SUPPORTING EACH OF THE 4 PILLARS OF MY HEALTH?

NUTRITION (NUTRIENT DENSE FOODS, WATER)

LIFESTYLE (SLEEP, STRESS MANAGEMENT, EXERCISE)

MINDSET (AFFIRMATIONS, KIND SELF TALK)

SUPPORT (ASK FOR HELP, REACH OUT TO A FRIEND)

TODAY'S DATE: ___/___/___

QUOTE OF THE DAY:

> *"Everything is figureoutable."*
> *— Marie Forleo*

TODAY I AM GRATEFUL FOR:

DAILY AFFIRMATION:
(WRITE ONCE AND REPEAT THROUGHOUT THE DAY)

> *I am not obligated to please people if it doesn't serve me.*

NOTES:

FOOD & SYMPTOM TRACKER:

TIME	FOOD	SYMPTOMS & MOOD CHANGES

HOW AM I SUPPORTING EACH OF THE 4 PILLARS OF MY HEALTH?

NUTRITION (NUTRIENT DENSE FOODS, WATER)

LIFESTYLE (SLEEP, STRESS MANAGEMENT, EXERCISE)

MINDSET (AFFIRMATIONS, KIND SELF TALK)

SUPPORT (ASK FOR HELP, REACH OUT TO A FRIEND)

TODAY'S DATE: ___/___/___

QUOTE OF THE DAY:

"I'm not a person who defends myself very often. I kind of let my actions speak for me." – Tom Brady

TODAY I AM GRATEFUL FOR:

DAILY AFFIRMATION:
(WRITE ONCE AND REPEAT THROUGHOUT THE DAY)

My desires are important and I am worthy of fulfilling them.

NOTES:

FOOD & SYMPTOM TRACKER:

TIME	FOOD	SYMPTOMS & MOOD CHANGES

HOW AM I SUPPORTING EACH OF THE 4 PILLARS OF MY HEALTH?

NUTRITION (NUTRIENT DENSE FOODS, WATER)

LIFESTYLE (SLEEP, STRESS MANAGEMENT, EXERCISE)

MINDSET (AFFIRMATIONS, KIND SELF TALK)

SUPPORT (ASK FOR HELP, REACH OUT TO A FRIEND)

TODAY'S DATE: ___/___/___

QUOTE OF THE DAY:

"What you give with an open heart is what returns."
— Jim Fortin

TODAY I AM GRATEFUL FOR:

DAILY AFFIRMATION:
(WRITE ONCE AND REPEAT THROUGHOUT THE DAY)

I face challenges head on.

NOTES:

FOOD & SYMPTOM TRACKER:

TIME	FOOD	SYMPTOMS & MOOD CHANGES

HOW AM I SUPPORTING EACH OF THE 4 PILLARS OF MY HEALTH?

NUTRITION (NUTRIENT DENSE FOODS, WATER)

LIFESTYLE (SLEEP, STRESS MANAGEMENT, EXERCISE)

MINDSET (AFFIRMATIONS, KIND SELF TALK)

SUPPORT (ASK FOR HELP, REACH OUT TO A FRIEND)

TODAY'S DATE: ___/___/___

QUOTE OF THE DAY:

> "Change is painful. Few people have the courage to seek out change. Most people won't change until the pain of where they are exceeds the pain of change." – Dave Ramsey

TODAY I AM GRATEFUL FOR:

DAILY AFFIRMATION:
(WRITE ONCE AND REPEAT THROUGHOUT THE DAY)

> I can do difficult things.

NOTES:

FOOD & SYMPTOM TRACKER:

TIME	FOOD	SYMPTOMS & MOOD CHANGES

HOW AM I SUPPORTING EACH OF THE 4 PILLARS OF MY HEALTH?

NUTRITION (NUTRIENT DENSE FOODS, WATER)

LIFESTYLE (SLEEP, STRESS MANAGEMENT, EXERCISE)

MINDSET (AFFIRMATIONS, KIND SELF TALK)

SUPPORT (ASK FOR HELP, REACH OUT TO A FRIEND)

TODAY'S DATE: ___/___/___

QUOTE OF THE DAY:

"If you think you are too small to make a difference, try sleeping with a mosquito." – Dalai Lama

TODAY I AM GRATEFUL FOR:

DAILY AFFIRMATION:
(WRITE ONCE AND REPEAT THROUGHOUT THE DAY)

Every day is a new opportunity to make my dreams come true.

NOTES:

FOOD & SYMPTOM TRACKER:

TIME	FOOD	SYMPTOMS & MOOD CHANGES

HOW AM I SUPPORTING EACH OF THE 4 PILLARS OF MY HEALTH?

NUTRITION (NUTRIENT DENSE FOODS, WATER)

LIFESTYLE (SLEEP, STRESS MANAGEMENT, EXERCISE)

MINDSET (AFFIRMATIONS, KIND SELF TALK)

SUPPORT (ASK FOR HELP, REACH OUT TO A FRIEND)

TODAY'S DATE: ___/___/___

QUOTE OF THE DAY:

"Be open to learning new lessons, even if they contradict the lessons you learned yesterday." — Ellen DeGeneres

TODAY I AM GRATEFUL FOR:

DAILY AFFIRMATION:
(WRITE ONCE AND REPEAT THROUGHOUT THE DAY)

My mind hears what my subconscious believes.

NOTES:

FOOD & SYMPTOM TRACKER:

TIME	FOOD	SYMPTOMS & MOOD CHANGES

HOW AM I SUPPORTING EACH OF THE 4 PILLARS OF MY HEALTH?

NUTRITION (NUTRIENT DENSE FOODS, WATER)

LIFESTYLE (SLEEP, STRESS MANAGEMENT, EXERCISE)

MINDSET (AFFIRMATIONS, KIND SELF TALK)

SUPPORT (ASK FOR HELP, REACH OUT TO A FRIEND)

TODAY'S DATE: ___/___/___

QUOTE OF THE DAY:

> "Have the courage to follow your heart and intuition. They somehow already know what you truly want to become." – Steve Jobs

TODAY I AM GRATEFUL FOR:

DAILY AFFIRMATION:
(WRITE ONCE AND REPEAT THROUGHOUT THE DAY)

> Money is an unlimited resource and I have total access to it.

NOTES:

FOOD & SYMPTOM TRACKER:

TIME	FOOD	SYMPTOMS & MOOD CHANGES

HOW AM I SUPPORTING EACH OF THE 4 PILLARS OF MY HEALTH?

NUTRITION (NUTRIENT DENSE FOODS, WATER)

LIFESTYLE (SLEEP, STRESS MANAGEMENT, EXERCISE)

MINDSET (AFFIRMATIONS, KIND SELF TALK)

SUPPORT (ASK FOR HELP, REACH OUT TO A FRIEND)

TODAY'S DATE: ___/___/___

QUOTE OF THE DAY:

"What we say to ourselves in the privacy of our own minds, matters. It drives our behavior, which drives our destiny, which shapes our world." – Marie Forleo

TODAY I AM GRATEFUL FOR:

DAILY AFFIRMATION:
(WRITE ONCE AND REPEAT THROUGHOUT THE DAY)

I am continuously healing and feeling better every day.

NOTES:

FOOD & SYMPTOM TRACKER:

TIME	FOOD	SYMPTOMS & MOOD CHANGES

HOW AM I SUPPORTING EACH OF THE 4 PILLARS OF MY HEALTH?

NUTRITION (NUTRIENT DENSE FOODS, WATER)

LIFESTYLE (SLEEP, STRESS MANAGEMENT, EXERCISE)

MINDSET (AFFIRMATIONS, KIND SELF TALK)

SUPPORT (ASK FOR HELP, REACH OUT TO A FRIEND)

TODAY'S DATE: ___/___/___

QUOTE OF THE DAY:

> "Optimism is the one quality more associated with success and happiness than any other." - Brian Tracy

TODAY I AM GRATEFUL FOR:

DAILY AFFIRMATION:
(WRITE ONCE AND REPEAT THROUGHOUT THE DAY)

> Today I am attracting new sources of money to come into my life.

NOTES:

FOOD & SYMPTOM TRACKER:

TIME	FOOD	SYMPTOMS & MOOD CHANGES

HOW AM I SUPPORTING EACH OF THE 4 PILLARS OF MY HEALTH?

NUTRITION (NUTRIENT DENSE FOODS, WATER)

LIFESTYLE (SLEEP, STRESS MANAGEMENT, EXERCISE)

MINDSET (AFFIRMATIONS, KIND SELF TALK)

SUPPORT (ASK FOR HELP, REACH OUT TO A FRIEND)

TODAY'S DATE: ___/___/___

QUOTE OF THE DAY:

"Yesterday I was clever, so I wanted to change the world. Today I am wise, so I am changing myself." – Rumi

TODAY I AM GRATEFUL FOR:

DAILY AFFIRMATION:
(WRITE ONCE AND REPEAT THROUGHOUT THE DAY)

Every feeling and emotion I have ever felt has been felt by someone before me.

NOTES:

FOOD & SYMPTOM TRACKER:

TIME	FOOD	SYMPTOMS & MOOD CHANGES

HOW AM I SUPPORTING EACH OF THE 4 PILLARS OF MY HEALTH?

NUTRITION (NUTRIENT DENSE FOODS, WATER)

LIFESTYLE (SLEEP, STRESS MANAGEMENT, EXERCISE)

MINDSET (AFFIRMATIONS, KIND SELF TALK)

SUPPORT (ASK FOR HELP, REACH OUT TO A FRIEND)

TODAY'S DATE: ___/___/___

QUOTE OF THE DAY:

> "Birds sing after a storm; why shouldn't people feel as free to delight in whatever sunlight remains to them?"
> – Rose Kennedy

TODAY I AM GRATEFUL FOR:

DAILY AFFIRMATION:
(WRITE ONCE AND REPEAT THROUGHOUT THE DAY)

> Today I will grow a little bit more into the person I am striving to become.

NOTES:

FOOD & SYMPTOM TRACKER:

TIME	FOOD	SYMPTOMS & MOOD CHANGES

HOW AM I SUPPORTING EACH OF THE 4 PILLARS OF MY HEALTH?

NUTRITION (NUTRIENT DENSE FOODS, WATER)

LIFESTYLE (SLEEP, STRESS MANAGEMENT, EXERCISE)

MINDSET (AFFIRMATIONS, KIND SELF TALK)

SUPPORT (ASK FOR HELP, REACH OUT TO A FRIEND)

TODAY'S DATE: ___/___/___

QUOTE OF THE DAY:

"If you do what you've always done, you'll get what you've always gotten." – Tony Robbins

TODAY I AM GRATEFUL FOR:

DAILY AFFIRMATION:
(WRITE ONCE AND REPEAT THROUGHOUT THE DAY)

I forgive myself because I deserve to be free.

NOTES:

FOOD & SYMPTOM TRACKER:

TIME	FOOD	SYMPTOMS & MOOD CHANGES

HOW AM I SUPPORTING EACH OF THE 4 PILLARS OF MY HEALTH?

NUTRITION (NUTRIENT DENSE FOODS, WATER)

LIFESTYLE (SLEEP, STRESS MANAGEMENT, EXERCISE)

MINDSET (AFFIRMATIONS, KIND SELF TALK)

SUPPORT (ASK FOR HELP, REACH OUT TO A FRIEND)

TODAY'S DATE: ___/___/___

QUOTE OF THE DAY:

"Once you figure out who you are and what you love about yourself, I think it all kinda falls into place."
— Jennifer Aniston

TODAY I AM GRATEFUL FOR:

DAILY AFFIRMATION:
(WRITE ONCE AND REPEAT THROUGHOUT THE DAY)

I am confident in the decisions I make because I am more than capable.

NOTES:

FOOD & SYMPTOM TRACKER:

TIME	FOOD	SYMPTOMS & MOOD CHANGES

HOW AM I SUPPORTING EACH OF THE 4 PILLARS OF MY HEALTH?

NUTRITION (NUTRIENT DENSE FOODS, WATER)

LIFESTYLE (SLEEP, STRESS MANAGEMENT, EXERCISE)

MINDSET (AFFIRMATIONS, KIND SELF TALK)

SUPPORT (ASK FOR HELP, REACH OUT TO A FRIEND)

TODAY'S DATE: ___/___/___

QUOTE OF THE DAY:

"Write it on your heart that every day is the best day in the year."
— Ralph Waldo Emerson

TODAY I AM GRATEFUL FOR:

DAILY AFFIRMATION:
(WRITE ONCE AND REPEAT THROUGHOUT THE DAY)

I am love and I am light.

NOTES:

FOOD & SYMPTOM TRACKER:

TIME	FOOD	SYMPTOMS & MOOD CHANGES

HOW AM I SUPPORTING EACH OF THE 4 PILLARS OF MY HEALTH?

NUTRITION (NUTRIENT DENSE FOODS, WATER)

LIFESTYLE (SLEEP, STRESS MANAGEMENT, EXERCISE)

MINDSET (AFFIRMATIONS, KIND SELF TALK)

SUPPORT (ASK FOR HELP, REACH OUT TO A FRIEND)

TODAY'S DATE: ___/___/___

QUOTE OF THE DAY:

> "I thank you God for this most amazing day, for the leaping greenly spirits of trees, and for the blue dream of sky and for everything which is natural, which is infinite, which is yes." - e.e. cummings

TODAY I AM GRATEFUL FOR:

DAILY AFFIRMATION:
(WRITE ONCE AND REPEAT THROUGHOUT THE DAY)

> I celebrate the good things that happen to those around me.

NOTES:

FOOD & SYMPTOM TRACKER:

TIME	FOOD	SYMPTOMS & MOOD CHANGES

HOW AM I SUPPORTING EACH OF THE 4 PILLARS OF MY HEALTH?

NUTRITION (NUTRIENT DENSE FOODS, WATER)

LIFESTYLE (SLEEP, STRESS MANAGEMENT, EXERCISE)

MINDSET (AFFIRMATIONS, KIND SELF TALK)

SUPPORT (ASK FOR HELP, REACH OUT TO A FRIEND)

TODAY'S DATE: ___/___/___

QUOTE OF THE DAY:

"What you get by achieving your goals is not as important as what you become by achieving your goals."
— Henry David Thoreau

TODAY I AM GRATEFUL FOR:

DAILY AFFIRMATION:
(WRITE ONCE AND REPEAT THROUGHOUT THE DAY)

I release what I cannot control.

NOTES:

FOOD & SYMPTOM TRACKER:

TIME	FOOD	SYMPTOMS & MOOD CHANGES

HOW AM I SUPPORTING EACH OF THE 4 PILLARS OF MY HEALTH?

NUTRITION (NUTRIENT DENSE FOODS, WATER)

LIFESTYLE (SLEEP, STRESS MANAGEMENT, EXERCISE)

MINDSET (AFFIRMATIONS, KIND SELF TALK)

SUPPORT (ASK FOR HELP, REACH OUT TO A FRIEND)

TODAY'S DATE: ___/___/___

QUOTE OF THE DAY:

"And suddenly you know: it's time to start something new and trust the magic of beginnings." - Meister Eckhart

TODAY I AM GRATEFUL FOR:

DAILY AFFIRMATION:
(WRITE ONCE AND REPEAT THROUGHOUT THE DAY)

I keep an open mind about concepts I don't understand.

NOTES:

FOOD & SYMPTOM TRACKER:

TIME	FOOD	SYMPTOMS & MOOD CHANGES

HOW AM I SUPPORTING EACH OF THE 4 PILLARS OF MY HEALTH?

NUTRITION (NUTRIENT DENSE FOODS, WATER)

LIFESTYLE (SLEEP, STRESS MANAGEMENT, EXERCISE)

MINDSET (AFFIRMATIONS, KIND SELF TALK)

SUPPORT (ASK FOR HELP, REACH OUT TO A FRIEND)

TODAY'S DATE: ___/___/___

QUOTE OF THE DAY:

"Never give up on a dream just because of the time it will take to accomplish it. The time will pass anyway." - Earl Nightingale

TODAY I AM GRATEFUL FOR:

DAILY AFFIRMATION:
(WRITE ONCE AND REPEAT THROUGHOUT THE DAY)

There is always something more to learn about a subject.

NOTES:

FOOD & SYMPTOM TRACKER:

TIME	FOOD	SYMPTOMS & MOOD CHANGES

HOW AM I SUPPORTING EACH OF THE 4 PILLARS OF MY HEALTH?

NUTRITION (NUTRIENT DENSE FOODS, WATER)

LIFESTYLE (SLEEP, STRESS MANAGEMENT, EXERCISE)

MINDSET (AFFIRMATIONS, KIND SELF TALK)

SUPPORT (ASK FOR HELP, REACH OUT TO A FRIEND)

TODAY'S DATE: ___/___/___

QUOTE OF THE DAY:

"Without leaps of imagination, or dreaming, we lose the excitement of possibilities. Dreaming, after all, is a form of planning." – Gloria Steinem

TODAY I AM GRATEFUL FOR:

DAILY AFFIRMATION:
(WRITE ONCE AND REPEAT THROUGHOUT THE DAY)

Today, amazing things are happening for me.

NOTES:

FOOD & SYMPTOM TRACKER:

TIME	FOOD	SYMPTOMS & MOOD CHANGES

HOW AM I SUPPORTING EACH OF THE 4 PILLARS OF MY HEALTH?

NUTRITION (NUTRIENT DENSE FOODS, WATER)

LIFESTYLE (SLEEP, STRESS MANAGEMENT, EXERCISE)

MINDSET (AFFIRMATIONS, KIND SELF TALK)

SUPPORT (ASK FOR HELP, REACH OUT TO A FRIEND)

TODAY'S DATE: ___/___/___

QUOTE OF THE DAY:

"Sometimes you win, sometimes you learn."
— John Maxwell

TODAY I AM GRATEFUL FOR:

DAILY AFFIRMATION:
(WRITE ONCE AND REPEAT THROUGHOUT THE DAY)

I always remember that challenges are temporary.

NOTES:

FOOD & SYMPTOM TRACKER:

TIME	FOOD	SYMPTOMS & MOOD CHANGES

HOW AM I SUPPORTING EACH OF THE 4 PILLARS OF MY HEALTH?

NUTRITION (NUTRIENT DENSE FOODS, WATER)

LIFESTYLE (SLEEP, STRESS MANAGEMENT, EXERCISE)

MINDSET (AFFIRMATIONS, KIND SELF TALK)

SUPPORT (ASK FOR HELP, REACH OUT TO A FRIEND)

TODAY'S DATE: ___/___/___

QUOTE OF THE DAY:

"Goals on the road to achievement cannot be achieved without discipline and consistency." - Denzel Washington

TODAY I AM GRATEFUL FOR:

DAILY AFFIRMATION:
(WRITE ONCE AND REPEAT THROUGHOUT THE DAY)

I am undeniably worthy of pure, whole joy and a fulfilled heart.

NOTES:

FOOD & SYMPTOM TRACKER:

TIME	FOOD	SYMPTOMS & MOOD CHANGES

HOW AM I SUPPORTING EACH OF THE 4 PILLARS OF MY HEALTH?

NUTRITION (NUTRIENT DENSE FOODS, WATER)

LIFESTYLE (SLEEP, STRESS MANAGEMENT, EXERCISE)

MINDSET (AFFIRMATIONS, KIND SELF TALK)

SUPPORT (ASK FOR HELP, REACH OUT TO A FRIEND)

TODAY'S DATE: ___/___/___

QUOTE OF THE DAY:

"The formula of happiness and success is just being actually yourself, in the most vivid possible way you can."
— Meryl Streep

TODAY I AM GRATEFUL FOR:

DAILY AFFIRMATION:
(WRITE ONCE AND REPEAT THROUGHOUT THE DAY)

I am capable of more than I know.

NOTES:

FOOD & SYMPTOM TRACKER:

TIME	FOOD	SYMPTOMS & MOOD CHANGES

HOW AM I SUPPORTING EACH OF THE 4 PILLARS OF MY HEALTH?

NUTRITION (NUTRIENT DENSE FOODS, WATER)

LIFESTYLE (SLEEP, STRESS MANAGEMENT, EXERCISE)

MINDSET (AFFIRMATIONS, KIND SELF TALK)

SUPPORT (ASK FOR HELP, REACH OUT TO A FRIEND)

TODAY'S DATE: ___/___/___

QUOTE OF THE DAY:

"Don't feel stupid if you don't like what everyone else pretends to love." – Emma Watson

TODAY I AM GRATEFUL FOR:

DAILY AFFIRMATION:
(WRITE ONCE AND REPEAT THROUGHOUT THE DAY)

I do not need all the answers to move forward.

NOTES:

FOOD & SYMPTOM TRACKER:

TIME	FOOD	SYMPTOMS & MOOD CHANGES

HOW AM I SUPPORTING EACH OF THE 4 PILLARS OF MY HEALTH?

NUTRITION (NUTRIENT DENSE FOODS, WATER)

LIFESTYLE (SLEEP, STRESS MANAGEMENT, EXERCISE)

MINDSET (AFFIRMATIONS, KIND SELF TALK)

SUPPORT (ASK FOR HELP, REACH OUT TO A FRIEND)

TODAY'S DATE: ___/___/___

QUOTE OF THE DAY:

"I will follow the upward road today. I will keep my face to the light. I will think high thoughts as I go my way. I will do what I know is right. I will look for the flowers by the side of the road. I will laugh and love and be strong. I will try to lighten another's load this day as I fare along." – Mary Susanne Edgar

TODAY I AM GRATEFUL FOR:

DAILY AFFIRMATION:
(WRITE ONCE AND REPEAT THROUGHOUT THE DAY)

I have patience for all the remarkable things coming my way.

NOTES:

FOOD & SYMPTOM TRACKER:

TIME	FOOD	SYMPTOMS & MOOD CHANGES

HOW AM I SUPPORTING EACH OF THE 4 PILLARS OF MY HEALTH?

NUTRITION (NUTRIENT DENSE FOODS, WATER)

LIFESTYLE (SLEEP, STRESS MANAGEMENT, EXERCISE)

MINDSET (AFFIRMATIONS, KIND SELF TALK)

SUPPORT (ASK FOR HELP, REACH OUT TO A FRIEND)

It's time to order a new journal!

Your "90-Day Self-Healing Journal" will end in two weeks. Order your next one now to keep up your momentum!

TODAY'S DATE: ___/___/___

QUOTE OF THE DAY:

"Laugh my friend, for laughter ignites a fire within the pit of your belly and awakens your being."
— Stella McCartney

TODAY I AM GRATEFUL FOR:

DAILY AFFIRMATION:
(WRITE ONCE AND REPEAT THROUGHOUT THE DAY)

I am safe here.

NOTES:

FOOD & SYMPTOM TRACKER:

TIME	FOOD	SYMPTOMS & MOOD CHANGES

HOW AM I SUPPORTING EACH OF THE 4 PILLARS OF MY HEALTH?

NUTRITION (NUTRIENT DENSE FOODS, WATER)

LIFESTYLE (SLEEP, STRESS MANAGEMENT, EXERCISE)

MINDSET (AFFIRMATIONS, KIND SELF TALK)

SUPPORT (ASK FOR HELP, REACH OUT TO A FRIEND)

TODAY'S DATE: ___/___/___

QUOTE OF THE DAY:

> *"Love what you do and do what you love. Don't listen to anyone else who tells you not to do it. You do what you want, what you love. Imagination should be the center of your life."* – Ray Bradbury

TODAY I AM GRATEFUL FOR:

DAILY AFFIRMATION:
(WRITE ONCE AND REPEAT THROUGHOUT THE DAY)

> *The world is good to me.*

NOTES:

FOOD & SYMPTOM TRACKER:

TIME	FOOD	SYMPTOMS & MOOD CHANGES

HOW AM I SUPPORTING EACH OF THE 4 PILLARS OF MY HEALTH?

NUTRITION (NUTRIENT DENSE FOODS, WATER)

LIFESTYLE (SLEEP, STRESS MANAGEMENT, EXERCISE)

MINDSET (AFFIRMATIONS, KIND SELF TALK)

SUPPORT (ASK FOR HELP, REACH OUT TO A FRIEND)

TODAY'S DATE: ___/___/___

QUOTE OF THE DAY:

"Know that you are the perfect age. Each year is special and precious, for you shall only live it once. Be comfortable with growing older." – Louise Hay

TODAY I AM GRATEFUL FOR:

DAILY AFFIRMATION:
(WRITE ONCE AND REPEAT THROUGHOUT THE DAY)

Today, I will give someone a hand, even if it seems like a small thing.

NOTES:

FOOD & SYMPTOM TRACKER:

TIME	FOOD	SYMPTOMS & MOOD CHANGES

HOW AM I SUPPORTING EACH OF THE 4 PILLARS OF MY HEALTH?

NUTRITION (NUTRIENT DENSE FOODS, WATER)

LIFESTYLE (SLEEP, STRESS MANAGEMENT, EXERCISE)

MINDSET (AFFIRMATIONS, KIND SELF TALK)

SUPPORT (ASK FOR HELP, REACH OUT TO A FRIEND)

TODAY'S DATE: ___/___/___

QUOTE OF THE DAY:

> "Your assumptions are your windows on the world. Scrub them off every once in a while, or the light won't come in." – Issac Asimov

TODAY I AM GRATEFUL FOR:

DAILY AFFIRMATION:
(WRITE ONCE AND REPEAT THROUGHOUT THE DAY)

> I laugh every day because it is medicine for my soul.

NOTES:

FOOD & SYMPTOM TRACKER:

TIME	FOOD	SYMPTOMS & MOOD CHANGES

HOW AM I SUPPORTING EACH OF THE 4 PILLARS OF MY HEALTH?

NUTRITION (NUTRIENT DENSE FOODS, WATER)

LIFESTYLE (SLEEP, STRESS MANAGEMENT, EXERCISE)

MINDSET (AFFIRMATIONS, KIND SELF TALK)

SUPPORT (ASK FOR HELP, REACH OUT TO A FRIEND)

TODAY'S DATE: __/__/__

QUOTE OF THE DAY:

"You are imperfect, you are wired for struggle, but you are worthy of love and belonging." - Brené Brown

TODAY I AM GRATEFUL FOR:

DAILY AFFIRMATION:
(WRITE ONCE AND REPEAT THROUGHOUT THE DAY)

Today I will smile at a stranger and spread kind human connection.

NOTES:

FOOD & SYMPTOM TRACKER:

TIME	FOOD	SYMPTOMS & MOOD CHANGES

HOW AM I SUPPORTING EACH OF THE 4 PILLARS OF MY HEALTH?

NUTRITION (NUTRIENT DENSE FOODS, WATER)

LIFESTYLE (SLEEP, STRESS MANAGEMENT, EXERCISE)

MINDSET (AFFIRMATIONS, KIND SELF TALK)

SUPPORT (ASK FOR HELP, REACH OUT TO A FRIEND)

TODAY'S DATE: ___/___/___

QUOTE OF THE DAY:

> "Often, people who can do, don't because they're afraid of what people that can't do will say about them doing." – Trevor Noah

TODAY I AM GRATEFUL FOR:

DAILY AFFIRMATION:
(WRITE ONCE AND REPEAT THROUGHOUT THE DAY)

> The thing I feel resistance towards is what I need to address.

NOTES:

FOOD & SYMPTOM TRACKER:

TIME	FOOD	SYMPTOMS & MOOD CHANGES

HOW AM I SUPPORTING EACH OF THE 4 PILLARS OF MY HEALTH?

NUTRITION (NUTRIENT DENSE FOODS, WATER)

LIFESTYLE (SLEEP, STRESS MANAGEMENT, EXERCISE)

MINDSET (AFFIRMATIONS, KIND SELF TALK)

SUPPORT (ASK FOR HELP, REACH OUT TO A FRIEND)

TODAY'S DATE: ___/___/___

QUOTE OF THE DAY:

"In nature, nothing is perfect and everything is perfect. Trees can be contorted, bent in weird ways, and they're still beautiful." — Alice Walker

TODAY I AM GRATEFUL FOR:

DAILY AFFIRMATION:
(WRITE ONCE AND REPEAT THROUGHOUT THE DAY)

I can choose to start over any day that I want to.

NOTES:

FOOD & SYMPTOM TRACKER:

TIME	FOOD	SYMPTOMS & MOOD CHANGES

HOW AM I SUPPORTING EACH OF THE 4 PILLARS OF MY HEALTH?

NUTRITION (NUTRIENT DENSE FOODS, WATER)

LIFESTYLE (SLEEP, STRESS MANAGEMENT, EXERCISE)

MINDSET (AFFIRMATIONS, KIND SELF TALK)

SUPPORT (ASK FOR HELP, REACH OUT TO A FRIEND)

TODAY'S DATE: ___/___/___

QUOTE OF THE DAY:

> "You must not lose faith in humanity. Humanity is like an ocean: if a few drops of the ocean are dirty, the ocean does not become dirty." - Mahatma Gandhi

TODAY I AM GRATEFUL FOR:

DAILY AFFIRMATION:
(WRITE ONCE AND REPEAT THROUGHOUT THE DAY)

> It is safe to take chances because most decisions are reversible or fixable.

NOTES:

FOOD & SYMPTOM TRACKER:

TIME	FOOD	SYMPTOMS & MOOD CHANGES

HOW AM I SUPPORTING EACH OF THE 4 PILLARS OF MY HEALTH?

NUTRITION (NUTRIENT DENSE FOODS, WATER)

LIFESTYLE (SLEEP, STRESS MANAGEMENT, EXERCISE)

MINDSET (AFFIRMATIONS, KIND SELF TALK)

SUPPORT (ASK FOR HELP, REACH OUT TO A FRIEND)

TODAY'S DATE: ___/___/___

QUOTE OF THE DAY:

"Never, ever, ever wear anything you are uncomfortable in. Because that is what you'll project: 'I look like a fool.' Even if you don't – you'll be tentative and not your best." – Tom Ford

TODAY I AM GRATEFUL FOR:

DAILY AFFIRMATION:
(WRITE ONCE AND REPEAT THROUGHOUT THE DAY)

I see beauty in even the most seemingly mundane moments.

NOTES:

FOOD & SYMPTOM TRACKER:

TIME	FOOD	SYMPTOMS & MOOD CHANGES

HOW AM I SUPPORTING EACH OF THE 4 PILLARS OF MY HEALTH?

NUTRITION (NUTRIENT DENSE FOODS, WATER)

LIFESTYLE (SLEEP, STRESS MANAGEMENT, EXERCISE)

MINDSET (AFFIRMATIONS, KIND SELF TALK)

SUPPORT (ASK FOR HELP, REACH OUT TO A FRIEND)

TODAY'S DATE: ___/___/___

QUOTE OF THE DAY:

"Those who cannot change their minds cannot change anything."
– George Bernard Shaw

TODAY I AM GRATEFUL FOR:

DAILY AFFIRMATION:
(WRITE ONCE AND REPEAT THROUGHOUT THE DAY)

I take one day at a time, because that's all I am ever given at once.

NOTES:

FOOD & SYMPTOM TRACKER:

TIME	FOOD	SYMPTOMS & MOOD CHANGES

HOW AM I SUPPORTING EACH OF THE 4 PILLARS OF MY HEALTH?

NUTRITION (NUTRIENT DENSE FOODS, WATER)

LIFESTYLE (SLEEP, STRESS MANAGEMENT, EXERCISE)

MINDSET (AFFIRMATIONS, KIND SELF TALK)

SUPPORT (ASK FOR HELP, REACH OUT TO A FRIEND)

TODAY'S DATE: ___/___/___

QUOTE OF THE DAY:

"Miracles do not, in fact, break the laws of nature." - C.S. Lewis

TODAY I AM GRATEFUL FOR:

DAILY AFFIRMATION:
(WRITE ONCE AND REPEAT THROUGHOUT THE DAY)

I do things outside of my comfort zone and each time I grow as a person.

NOTES:

FOOD & SYMPTOM TRACKER:

TIME	FOOD	SYMPTOMS & MOOD CHANGES

HOW AM I SUPPORTING EACH OF THE 4 PILLARS OF MY HEALTH?

NUTRITION (NUTRIENT DENSE FOODS, WATER)

LIFESTYLE (SLEEP, STRESS MANAGEMENT, EXERCISE)

MINDSET (AFFIRMATIONS, KIND SELF TALK)

SUPPORT (ASK FOR HELP, REACH OUT TO A FRIEND)

TODAY'S DATE: ___/___/___

QUOTE OF THE DAY:

> "You, yourself, as much as anybody in the entire universe, deserve your love and affection." - Buddah

TODAY I AM GRATEFUL FOR:

DAILY AFFIRMATION:
(WRITE ONCE AND REPEAT THROUGHOUT THE DAY)

> I am wholly loved and cherished. I matter.

NOTES:

FOOD & SYMPTOM TRACKER:

TIME	FOOD	SYMPTOMS & MOOD CHANGES

HOW AM I SUPPORTING EACH OF THE 4 PILLARS OF MY HEALTH?

NUTRITION (NUTRIENT DENSE FOODS, WATER)

LIFESTYLE (SLEEP, STRESS MANAGEMENT, EXERCISE)

MINDSET (AFFIRMATIONS, KIND SELF TALK)

SUPPORT (ASK FOR HELP, REACH OUT TO A FRIEND)

TODAY'S DATE: ___/___/___

QUOTE OF THE DAY:

"The pessimist sees difficulty in every opportunity. The optimist sees opportunity in every difficulty." – Winston Churchill

TODAY I AM GRATEFUL FOR:

DAILY AFFIRMATION:
(WRITE ONCE AND REPEAT THROUGHOUT THE DAY)

My time is precious and I use it wisely.

NOTES:

FOOD & SYMPTOM TRACKER:

TIME	FOOD	SYMPTOMS & MOOD CHANGES

HOW AM I SUPPORTING EACH OF THE 4 PILLARS OF MY HEALTH?

NUTRITION (NUTRIENT DENSE FOODS, WATER)

LIFESTYLE (SLEEP, STRESS MANAGEMENT, EXERCISE)

MINDSET (AFFIRMATIONS, KIND SELF TALK)

SUPPORT (ASK FOR HELP, REACH OUT TO A FRIEND)

TODAY'S DATE: ___/___/___

QUOTE OF THE DAY:

> *"I attribute my success to this: I never gave or took any excuse."*
> *—Florence Nightingale*

TODAY I AM GRATEFUL FOR:

DAILY AFFIRMATION:
(WRITE ONCE AND REPEAT THROUGHOUT THE DAY)

> *I have faith in my future.*
> *I have faith in me.*

NOTES:

FOOD & SYMPTOM TRACKER:

TIME	FOOD	SYMPTOMS & MOOD CHANGES

HOW AM I SUPPORTING EACH OF THE 4 PILLARS OF MY HEALTH?

NUTRITION (NUTRIENT DENSE FOODS, WATER)

LIFESTYLE (SLEEP, STRESS MANAGEMENT, EXERCISE)

MINDSET (AFFIRMATIONS, KIND SELF TALK)

SUPPORT (ASK FOR HELP, REACH OUT TO A FRIEND)

Congratulations!

You have finished 90 days of goal setting and tracking, and now it's time to come full circle and evaluate your goals.

My nutrition goal for the next 90 days was:

What did I do well? How could I improve this goal?

My mindset goal for the next 90 days was:

What did I do well? How could I improve this goal?

My support goal for the next 90 days was:

What did I do well? How could I improve this goal?

My lifestyle goal for the next 90 days was:

What did I do well? How could I improve this goal?

Don't forget to order your next 90-Day Self-Healing Journal to get ready for another 90 days of growth and healing on Amazon.

Please send questions, comments, and greetings to alexa@girlinhealing.com.

"She will not worry, she will be just fine. She will brave the new season one day at a time."

– Morgan Harper Nichols

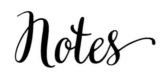

Made in the USA
San Bernardino, CA
24 March 2020

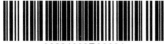